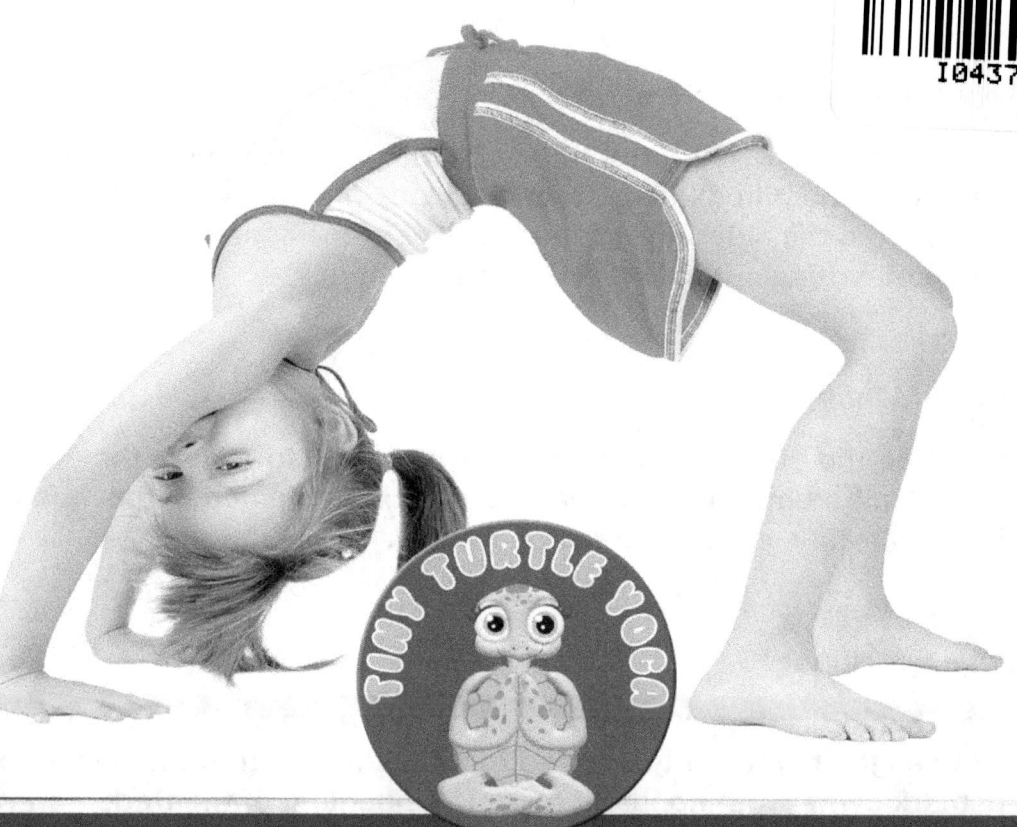

BREATHE · MOVE · LEARN · PLAY

TINY TURTLE
YOGA GUIDE

Answers to your questions
about Kids Yoga and Yoga

By Alicia Chapman Mauldin
RYT-200, RCYT, CYKT

Disclaimers / Legal Information

All rights reserved. No part of this book may be reproduced, stored in a retrieval system, or transmitted in any form or by any means, without the prior written permission of the author/publisher, except in the case of brief quotations for the purpose of writing critical articles or reviews.

Notice of Liability

The author and publisher have made every effort to ensure the accuracy of the information herein. However, the information contained in this book is presented without warranty, either express or implied.

Trademark Notice

Rather than indicating every occurrence of a trademarked name as such, this book uses the names only in an editorial fashion and to the benefit of the trademark owner with no intention of infringement of the trademark.

Copyright Information

©2014 Jack Quinn Solutions, LLC

About Alicia

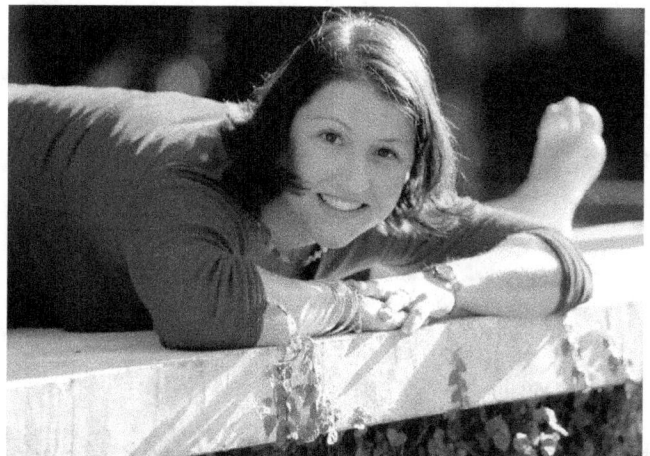

Alicia Mauldin, RYT-200, RCYT, CYKT

Alicia Chapman Mauldin graduated from the University of Florida with a degree in Business. With a background in dance instruction, she naturally fell in love with yoga. It did not take long before she followed her passion for instructing, and began teaching yoga classes. She has been teaching yoga since 2002 and brings a playful personality to her regular adult yoga classes.

Alicia is a mother of three young children. She wanted to share the joys of yoga with more than her own children, and began teaching kids' yoga classes in 2010. She trained with YogaKids and is a Registered Children's Yoga Teacher with Yoga Alliance. Alicia has a passion for teaching & training, and enjoys sharing her knowledge with others. She is also the Mentor Coordinator for YogaKids International, inspiring and motivating the students currently training with YogaKids. Alicia likes to laugh and keep yoga fun for both adults and children.

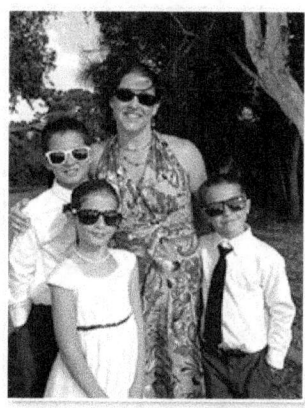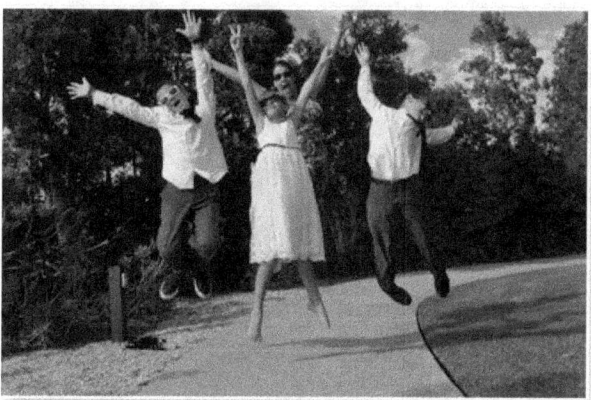

My mission is to teach children how to listen to their inner voice, appreciate their surroundings, and gain tools for dealing with life's challenges in a fun, non-competitive environment. Tiny Turtle Yoga classes for kids benefits children's minds, bodies, and spirits, while focusing on the whole child and teaching them to experience the joy in yoga. My mission is to teach yoga, educate others about yoga, and enjoy yoga every day!

Learn More...

As life presents many challenges to children these days, they can learn how to navigate their world in a positive way. Not only will yoga help children be physically healthier, it also helps their mental and emotional well-being. They learn how to control their energies and manage stress levels. They learn about their bodies, relationships with others, and the importance of self-talk. They also begin to identify and establish their place in this world. With these tools, children can grow up with more awareness, compassion, and joy.

To learn how yoga can help your family, visit http://www.yogaformykids.com to get a FREE Yoga Guide to Energy Strategies For Kids where you can learn the yoga movements and breathing exercises to help energize, focus, or calm your child. PLUS, you get access to our videos that demonstrate each move.

Contents

TINY TURTLE YOGA GUIDE

(Answers to your questions about Kids' Yoga and Yoga)

By Alicia Chapman Mauldin

RYT-200, RCYT, CYKT

Part 1: KIDS' YOGA

What is yoga exactly?

What are the benefits of kids' yoga?

How is kids' yoga different from Adult yoga?

How do Tiny Turtle yoga classes differ from other kids' yoga classes?

Who is qualified to teach yoga to kids?

How important are the specified age groups for a kid's yoga class?

What if my child just sits there and does not participate in the class?

How do children learn through yoga?

When can a child use yoga throughout their day?

How can yoga help my child be a better student?

How can yoga help children control their emotions?

How can yoga help my child athlete?

How can yoga help my child sleep better?

How does yoga help children with special needs?

How will yoga help my child grow to be a well-balanced adult?

Part 2: YOGA PHILOSOPHIES

Is yoga religious?

When did yoga come to the West?

What are the 8 limbs of yoga?

Why are so many yogis vegetarians?

What is karma yoga?

What does Om mean?

Why do people chant during yoga?

What is a mantra?

What is a mudra?

What are the chakras?

What does Namasté mean?

Part 3: YOGA CLASSES

Who can practice yoga?

What are the benefits of practicing yoga?

What are the different styles of yoga?

Which style of yoga should I practice?

What do I need for a yoga class?

Is there yoga class etiquette?

Why is yoga practiced barefoot?

How long are yoga classes?

How long do I wait after eating before practicing yoga?

Are all yoga teachers the same?

Would I benefit from a private yoga session?

Why do some yoga students use props?

Do I need to be flexible to practice yoga?

How is yoga breathing different from my normal breath?

How can yoga help me reduce stress?

What do the yoga certifications mean?

Why do people get hurt while practicing yoga?

What can I expect to do during a yoga class?

Why do yogis look like they are sleeping at the end of class?

What is the purpose of guided visualizations?

How often should I practice yoga?

Can I practice yoga at home?

When should I start practicing yoga?

Part 1- KIDS' YOGA

What is yoga?

When you hear the word "yoga," you may think of a person in a very twisted pose requiring a ridiculous amount of flexibility, or you may picture a person seated in a quiet meditation pose chanting the word "Om." Though these two people are practicing advanced aspects of yoga, there is so much more to yoga that makes it accessible to everyone, every age, every size, and every capability.

Yoga is a 4,000-year-old-philosophy, which includes physical postures, breathing exercises, meditation, and one's moral actions in a desire to reach enlightenment; pure of heart and full of joy. Part Two of this Yoga Guide explains more about yoga philosophies, answering questions about Om, Namasté, and why many yogis are vegetarians. Part Three discusses yoga classes, including class etiquette, differences between yoga styles, what to expect during a yoga class, and much more. Many people just practice the "exercise" component of yoga, but when the philosophies of yoga are also introduced to one's life, the benefits far exceed doing splits and handstands!

What are the benefits of kids' yoga?

Kids can benefit from yoga, just like adults. Physically, yoga helps increase strength, flexibility, balance, coordination, imagination, and the ability to control stress. Yoga is unique in that it uses one's own body weight and effort as resistance, so every child can do it. Yoga poses and breathing exercises help to calm kids, focus them, or energize them. As children practice yoga, they learn how to better control their emotions. When educational concepts are added to movements with their bodies, learning not only becomes fun, it also increases children's retention rates. Yoga also focuses on the breath; relaxing the nervous system and helping children feel better physically and mentally. In yoga, everyone is welcomed and accepted. Doesn't it sound amazing?

How is kids' yoga different from adult yoga?

Though many of the poses are similar to adult yoga, kids' yoga classes include the "fun" element. While in a Downward Facing Dog pose, for example, kids may bark like dogs or run their feet. There is less concern about form and alignment, as long as the child is safe, their pose is just right! Kids' yoga is about positivity, engagement, and learning about the body. Kids' yoga classes are not quiet! In addition to noises, kids' classes often involve interaction between the teacher and students or the students with each other. The teacher may ask, "What color is your butterfly?" while the students are holding the butterfly pose, and the children take turns answering. This enables the children to hold the poses longer and be engaged in the class.

Kids' yoga classes often have a theme. It may be for a specific holiday such as the 4th of July, or a general theme like "a day at the circus." In addition to practicing poses related to the theme, there are often games promoting cooperation, partner poses encouraging teamwork, and crafts to foster creativity. The possibilities are limitless!

How do Tiny Turtle Yoga classes differ from other kids' yoga classes?

After 10 years of teaching yoga to adults and having three children, I knew there was more to kids' yoga than teaching adult poses to little people. When I tried to teach regular poses to kids (even with a fun theme), the children lost interest and were bored. I decided to train with YogaKids in 2012 and began teaching kids' yoga classes the "YogaKids way." As described in *YogaKids: Educating the whole child through yoga* by Marsha Wenig, YogaKids is about teaching the child through movement and their kinesthetic body. YogaKids acknowledges that children process information through a variety of ways (music, math, reading, games, environment, etc.). By integrating different elements of learning into a yoga class, the children are engaged while moving their bodies and learning all at the same time. They leave yoga class feeling better and knowing more!

As a registered yoga teacher for adults, I have the knowledge and experience to sequence a well-balanced class for kids which is also fun and interactive. Classes begin with an opening circle to discuss the theme and get to know each other, followed by some warm up poses and the lesson plan. Towards the end of class, there may be cooperative games, arts and crafts, quiet time, journaling, or other activities to teach the child about the many benefits of yoga. Children love Tiny Turtle Yoga classes because they are accepted and feel successful. I have a student who is not very athletic and is not comfortable playing soccer or other sports at school, but at yoga she is always a winner.

Who is qualified to teach yoga to kids?

You! Anyone who has children in their lives can teach them yoga! As a parent, grandparent, or caregiver, you can learn simple yoga poses or breathing exercises and do them with children. Adults benefit from yoga too, so practice yoga with the child in your life, so you both enjoy the benefits! A teacher can introduce certain yoga concepts in a classroom to help calm rowdy children, focus their minds before a test, or ignite creativity before a writing assignment.

If attending a live kids' yoga class, the instructor should have experience with both yoga and yoga for children. There are a few programs available which offer workshops and trainings for those wishing to learn how to teach yoga to children. Yoga Alliance has established the standard for a 95-hour training program to distinguish yoga teachers certified to teach yoga to children. Upon completion, they receive the designation of Registered Children's Yoga Teacher (RCYT) in addition to their Registered Yoga Teacher (RYT) designation.

You do not need to be a certified yoga teacher to teach yoga to children. The 95 hour programs are generally open to the public, training educators, physical or occupational therapists, counselors, or volunteers who work with children. Each individual program may offer its own certification as well. For example, as a graduate of the YogaKids program, I am also a Certified YogaKids Teacher (CYKT). You can search YogaKids.com for a certified teacher near you on their "find a teacher" page.

How important are the specified age groups for a kid's yoga class?

Different yoga teachers will usually suggest an appropriate age for a particular kids' yoga class. In order for the class to be age appropriate for your child, respect the suggested age group because class length, poses practiced, instructions given, and activities planned are different for each age group. For example, if a preschooler attends a class intended for older students, the class may be too long and not include enough movement.

If the class is geared towards preschoolers, or those under the age of 6, the class will typically be shorter (maybe 30 minutes) due to their shorter attention spans, and should include lots of movement and pretend play. The poses are often simple to execute, with little direction, and there is not a lot of left versus right instruction. Simple letters, sounds, numbers, and fun animal facts may be introduced. There might be a story related to the theme of the day, but the children are invited to move along with the story and act it out (and not necessarily sit and listen). Quiet time may contain breathing exercises, guided visualizations, or a minute or two of resting in relaxation pose.

School aged children can enjoy a longer class, 45-60 minutes. These classes will likely include more challenging poses, which may be are held for longer periods of time. They love to answer questions, so they should have plenty of opportunities to share with the group. This age group loves trying new things, so classes should include a variety of activities, and they welcome ideas they can repeat at home. Educational content can be more age appropriate, including math facts and related science lessons. This age group loves stories too, but the moral of the story can have deeper meanings prompting conversations. Games, partner poses, and crafts are always a big hit, allowing them to take what they have learned in class and absorb the information in a different way. Quiet time can be longer, and more time can be spent in relaxation pose. Through a guided relaxation exercise, children are able to relax and be entertained at the same time. The more they practice relaxation, the more comfortable they get with it and the more they like it. Sometimes children need to experience a relaxation pose 6-8 times before they truly embrace the concept of being still and quiet.

Pre-teens and teens are almost ready for an adult class (though they can physically do it, they may still get bored). This is where a registered yoga teacher who also teaches kids can have a lot of fun. The poses are structured much like an adult class, but with the ability to reach out to teens instilling non-judgment, non-competition, acceptance, and teamwork. Teens are ready to learn more about proper alignment and how to do more challenging yoga poses (like they see in magazines). They still want to have fun so they may enjoy playing games and practicing partner poses, strengthening their interpersonal skills. Teens have so much to deal with in today's world, so yoga class becomes an opportunity to express themselves through discussions or journaling. A kid's yoga class teacher will take all of this into account when planning their lessons to ensure they are appropriate for the intended students. The age group suggested for the class should be followed to ensure your child has the best yoga experience possible.

What if my child just sits there and does not participate in the class?

Yoga should be a safe space and neither the teacher nor the parent should force a child to participate. Some young personalities are hesitant to jump in and try something new, such as a kids' yoga class. Don't be worried if your child sits on their mat and watches the entire class, instead of participating. They may enjoy watching the show! You will be surprised how much they are retaining. Those children can usually tell their parents every pose and activity from the class, and even practice it themselves at home. Once they get more comfortable with the teacher, environment, and other students, they usually join right in! They are still learning and receiving many benefits from watching.

Children have off days just like adults do. If they are not feeling themselves, are upset about something, and are not in the right space for yoga that day, they may need to have some quiet time on their mat. This might be just what they need at that particular moment. Teaching kids to listen to their bodies and respond to their immediate needs enables them to self-regulate their emotions. If a child needs a break from an activity, they should be able to take it. They typically rejoin the group when they are ready and are welcomed back with a smile.

How do children learn through yoga?

Based on Howard Gardner's theory of multiple intelligences, there are eight different ways information is processed: verbal, logical, visual, body, musical, with others, within oneself, and through nature. The more ways information is presented, the more it is retained. Tiny Turtle Yoga classes introduce information through many of the different intelligences during a yoga class, enabling children to connect with the information in a way that makes sense to them. While working with a homeschool group, I was able to take the lessons for the week and adapt yoga poses and games to teach or reinforce concepts. In a recent class, the children acted out the water cycle, held poses while counting by 6's to work on their math facts, and discussed the importance of taking care of our planet. By involving movement, the information is stored in the cells of the body for later retrieval.

According to the Learning Pyramid, we only retain 10% of what we read, 20% of what we hear, 30% of what we watch, 50% of discussion, 75% of what we do, and 90% of what we teach others (source: National Training Laboratories, Bethel, Maine). A typical classroom usually delivers information in a passive way (lecture, reading, demonstration). In order to increase student retention rates, they need to get involved by participating in discussions, moving their kinesthetic bodies, or teaching others.

When can a child use yoga throughout their day?

Yoga poses can help calm, energize, or focus children's energy. When my daughter gets upset at school, she takes a trip to the restroom, where she can take 5 deep breaths to calm herself down before returning to her desk. If a little sluggish in the morning or after lunchtime, there are poses and breathing exercises that can help children oxygenate the brain and awaken the body; like the Shake Like Jelly pose to move all the joints and muscles or bending forward to help send oxygen rich blood to the brain. To help focus and concentrate before tackling homework, balancing on one leg or having the arms and/or legs crisscross the body is a great way to get the brain engaged. As children learn techniques during yoga classes, they can apply those skills to their daily lives, self-regulating their energy for a more successful outcome.

How can yoga help my child be a better student?

Children naturally want to be upside down, but kids today are not climbing trees and hanging from the monkey bars like they used to. In yoga, kids get the opportunity to take the head below the heart and be upside down again! This oxygenates the brain and calms the nervous system. When children are both alert and relaxed, they are in the optimal state for learning. Let me say that again—both alert AND relaxed! If a child learns how to achieve these two things at the same time, they can improve their ability to learn and retain information. I suggest to my children that, before a test or challenging concept, they should bend over and retie their shoes (to be less conspicuous). This will help send fresh oxygen to their brain and help them be better thinkers. They also know some simple poses that help the left and right sides of the brain communicate, to better focus the mind. They might stand on one foot, cross the mid-line of their body with their arms or legs (giving themselves a hug, or pretending to scratch their back), or look up/down and left/right with their eyes to help activate the different parts of the brain. The Learning Station has some great songs on their Brain Boogie Boosters album, with videos featuring Tiny Turtle Yoga!

How can yoga help children control their emotions?

Since different yoga poses and breathing exercises affect our nervous systems, they alter our different energies. Children can learn techniques to handle their own stress levels. Just as adults respond to stress differently, so do children. Children can use the same principles adults use to alter their stressful state with different yoga poses and breathing exercises. The Child's Pose (on your knees, belly to your thighs, and forehead on the ground) is a great calming yoga pose, followed by long, deep, and even breaths to calm the nervous system. Practicing a small yoga series during the day leaves a child feeling refreshed and relaxed. If a child is agitated or upset, they are not going to learn the presented information. Having these tools can help teachers and parents redirect the energy of a child to get back to an optimal learning state. It is like a little magical yoga wand!

How can yoga help my child athlete?

Yoga is a great way to warm up the body before playing sports. The Sun Salutation is a series of poses (including Forward Folds, Lunges, Planks, Upward Facing Dog, and Downward Facing Dog) designed to move all of the muscles and joints of the body, a great pre-practice warm up. If your child plays soccer and will be running a lot, their warm up should not be more of the same movement, it should instead prepare the body for a practice or game; Warrior poses, Lunges, and Squats might be more appropriate.

When a child finds a sport they like, they tend to do it a lot. The problem with athletes that do the same sport or activity repetitively is that they often over train the muscle groups that help them excel in their sport but neglect others. This creates imbalance in their bodies. As certain muscles get stronger (thighs), without concern for the opposing muscle group (hamstrings), the muscles pull on the joints and create instability, which can lead to joint pain or even injury. I recently worked with some 8 and -9-year-old girls, on a competitive soccer team who were already experiencing knee pain from intense training. Focusing on strength and flexibility of the muscles supporting the joints will help those girls become faster and more powerful.

Becoming aware of the power of the breath is also very important for athletes. As they get nervous and adrenaline levels rise, their body is in a stressed state and does not use its energy efficiently. Learning to control the breath, calm the nervous system, and oxygenate the muscles will not only help give your athlete a clear head, it will also improve their endurance as they use their energy more efficiently. Working with a qualified yoga instructor, to tailor a yoga program for your young athlete, can help them prevent injury, build strength and flexibility, and improve their mental game.

How can yoga help my child sleep better?

Taking long, deep, full, and complete breaths can help calm the nervous system and prepare the body for sleep. Refer back to the question about yoga breathing for more information about the benefits of deep breathing. There are also certain calming poses that are great to do before bedtime; seated forward folds and legs up the wall are a few of my favorites.

Guided visualizations are also useful for children. Some wonderful examples are in the book *Spinning Inward* by Maureen Murdock. There are multiple exercises for all ages. If a child is having trouble sleeping because they are worried about something, a visualization exercise may help them release that worry. They can imagine placing that worrisome item in a basket and attaching it to a balloon. As the balloon flies away, it takes their worry with it and the child can visualize letting it go and feeling relieved.

How does yoga help children with special needs?

In yoga class, everyone is equal; everyone is a star and everyone wins. With a focus on acceptance and positive affirmations, children feel empowered and successful afterwards. Yoga gives all children, including those with special needs, tools they can use every day to help them communicate, relate to others, and deal with their emotions. It also helps improve focus, balance, strength, and flexibility in a cooperative, non-judgmental way—unlike any other sport or exercise. Yoga also allows children to find variations of poses that are physically possible for their body type. My favorite aspect of teaching yoga to kids is reminding them about the power of self-talk. By adding affirmations such as, "I am strong," or "I am confident," to poses, it connects our feelings with an action, and helps the body absorb and believe the statement. When children have the opportunity to verbally share these affirmations with the rest of the class, it gives them confidence and an opportunity to say something nice about themselves and feel good about it.

How will yoga help my child grow up to be a well-balanced adult?

As life presents many challenges to children these days, they can learn how to navigate their world in a positive way. Not only will yoga help children be physically healthier, it also helps their mental and emotional well-being. They learn how to control their energies and manage stress levels. They learn about their bodies, relationships with others, and the importance of self-talk. They also begin to identify and establish their place in this world. With these tools, children can grow up with more awareness, compassion, and joy. To quote Marsha Wenig, founder of YogaKids, "If kids are our future, shouldn't they be YogaKids?"

Part 2 - YOGA PHILOSOPHIES

Is yoga religious?

Yoga has been practiced in India for more than 4000 years. The original yogis (one who practices yoga) removed themselves from society and went into caves to meditate in search of enlightenment. There are stories that yogis would become stiff and uncomfortable after sitting and meditating for long periods of time, so they began to bend, twist, stretch, and move to keep their muscles and joints supple, enabling them to meditate for longer periods of time. There was not a formal yoga class, just individuals moving and breathing to help prepare their minds and bodies for lengthy meditations.

Two thousand years ago, the sage Patanjali compiled the Yoga Sutras, 195 statements of yoga practices and theories. He was the creator of the 8 limbs of yoga, suggesting not only that postures and meditation will lead to everlasting contentment, but also change attitudes and behaviors. Though yoga is not a religion, it is quite spiritual. It is exactly what it needs to be for the person practicing it. Through the moral actions of being a good person (a common thread in many religions), and practicing the ability to let go of external chatter and listen to one's inner voice, practicing yoga will enable a person to become more connected and spiritual (in their own faith). Since yoga originated in India, it is often associated with the Hindu religion, but yoga existed a long time before organized religion. Some religions adopted aspects of yoga as part of their worship or faith, not the other way around. Yoga acknowledges a higher power but does not identify who or what that is, since it is different for each of us. This aspect of yoga is about connecting with yourself and deepening your personal spirituality, no matter your religion.

When did yoga come to the West?

Westerners discovered yoga less than a century ago and are most familiar with "Hatha Yoga," poses and breathing exercises in particular. The current yoga trend gives little attention to the first limbs of yoga (be a good person and do good things) or to the upper limbs of yoga (concentration, meditation, and bliss). Of course, there are physical benefits to just practicing the physical poses in a yoga class, since they move every muscle and joint in the body, improving strength, flexibility, and balance. Practicing breathing control is something everyone should learn to help reduce daily stress, think more clearly, and relax the mind and body. In yoga, there is no competition or judgment. So if you attend a yoga class for merely the physical benefits, keep the spirit of yoga philosophies in mind. Others may be there for a different purpose (practicing the 8 limbs of yoga and living the 4 paths of yoga), to become a better person inside and out. But be careful; yoga has a way of opening your heart and clearing your mind, and you might find yourself desiring to be a better person with more love and acceptance off your yoga mat!

What are the 8 limbs of yoga?

Yoga is the Sanksrit word for "yuj" meaning to join or unite. Yoga is a philosophy, a way of living and interacting with the world. The physical practice of yoga integrates the mind, body, and breath. When you do yoga poses, you should move consciously, being aware of the body, and link your movements with your breath. As the body and the mind are better connected, one's physiological state begins to shift. The stress response in the body is overridden and the levels of the stress hormone (cortisol) in the blood stream are lowered. This helps create a clear slate to develop mental focus, strength, balance, and flexibility.

The philosophies of yoga are more than 4,000 years old; and, about 2,000 years ago, the sage Patanjali outlined the 8 limbs of yoga. Limbs 1-5 address an individual's relationship with the external world and limbs 6-8 are about one's relationship with oneself. Through this progressive series of practices, we strive to reach the eighth limb, but we all must start with the first. These 8 limbs can be visualized and detailed in the physical aspects of a tree.

The first limb is at the base of the tree – the roots, our principles to live by – called the Yamas. These are often referred to as the "DON'Ts" in our lives. Don't harm (be kind to others in words and actions); don't lie (tell the truth); don't steal (take only what is yours); don't have excess (practice moderation), and don't be greedy (share). The second limb is the trunk of the tree – our personal disciplines – called the Niyamas. These are the "DO's". Do be pure and clean; do practice acceptance; do your work; do take time to reflect, and Do stay humble. These first two limbs are the foundation of yoga. Be a good person and be good to others. Doesn't this sound nice? If everyone just practiced the first two limbs of yoga, the world would be filled with so much more goodness, compassion, and joy.

The next three limbs are more familiar aspects of yoga. These three limbs collectively comprise "Hatha Yoga," the physical practice of yoga. Most physical yoga classes in the Western world fall under the umbrella of Hatha yoga. "Ha" means sun and is our masculine or strong energy. "Tha" means moon and is our feminine or gentle energy. Everyone has both masculine and feminine energies. Physical yoga practice is about balancing these two energies through particular movements and breathing exercises. There are many different stylized yoga classes, moving at different paces, different intensities, different emphases, and even different temperatures. Some examples are Vinyasa, Iyengar, Ashtanga, Bikram, and Yin. Further explanation about these styles and more can be found in Part 3, "What are the different styles of yoga?"

The third limb is the yoga postures (called Asana), represented by strong yet flexible branches. This is what we most frequently associate with yoga. Imagine flexible branches, bending and twisting, without breaking. This is how we want our bodies to feel after practicing yoga poses and for the rest of our lives. Yoga poses should feel good. They should never hurt or leave us feeling worse than we did before class. The fourth limb is breath control (called Pranayama) and is represented by the breathing green leaves of a tree. The focus on the breath is an important practice in yoga, as our breath controls our "prana" or life energy. The postures and breathing exercises are meant to help balance the energies of the body and calm the mind, in preparation for practicing the next limbs of yoga. The fifth limb of the yoga tree is sense withdrawal (called Pratyahara). Drawing our attention inward and letting go of external distractions helps us to listen to the subtle messages of the body. This is the bark of the tree, protecting the tree from outside elements and preventing its essence from flowing outward.

After living the first two limbs of yoga (principles and disciplines) and practicing the three limbs of Hatha Yoga (postures, breath control, and sense withdrawal), the mind and body are prepared to practice the last three limbs of the yoga tree. Deep concentration (called Dharana) is the sixth limb of yoga, and is represented by the sap of the tree running through its veins and leaves, keeping the body-mind firm and connected. Staying with a focused state of concentration is Meditation (called Dhyana), the seventh limb, represented by a flower, the slow ripening of our consciousness. After all the other limbs have been practiced, ultimate meditation leads to pure bliss. Self-realization (called Samadhi) is the eighth and final limb of the tree, represented by the fullest fruit. At this point, our intentions are pure and our hearts and souls are full. Some yogis may never reach this final limb; but they may live, practice, breathe, concentrate, and meditate in hopes of experiencing pure bliss in their lifetime.

Why are so many yogis vegetarians?

On the first limb of the yoga tree, one of the yoga principles to live by is to "do no harm" (be kind to others). Many yogis apply this to all of the animals on the earth. They do not eat meat, since it certainly harms the animal. Not all people who practice yoga are vegetarians, but as yogis deepen their practice and embrace its principles and disciplines, they often move in the direction of more conscious eating.

What is karma yoga?

You may think of karma as doing good things for others and good things will come your way, and vice versa. According to a classic yoga text (*the Bhagavad Gita*), there are four paths of yoga, and karma yoga is one of those paths. No path is entirely separate from the others and can be compared to the body of a bird in flight.

The first path is called **Raja yoga (royal),** the "yoga of practice," and is associated with the head of the bird, providing guidance, vision, and organization. Raja yoga has 8 different elements one should practice regularly, including principles to live by, personal disciplines, postures, breath control, sense withdrawal, concentration, meditation, and ultimately self-realization.

The wings and tail of the bird are the "yoga of life," integrating yoga philosophies and actions into our daily lives. One of the wings of the bird is **Karma yoga (action),** the yoga of service. Karma yoga is performing truly selfless acts without the need or desire for compensation or recognition. The key to karma yoga is selflessness, doing good things, and serving others when no one is looking or will know to acknowledge it. **Bhakti yoga (faithfulness),** the yoga of devotion, is the other wing of the bird, representing our love, faith, and surrender. It is through our faith in people and a higher power that we are guided to move through life and its challenges. The tail of the bird is **Jñana yoga (knowledge**), yoga of life study. The study of philosophy, life, and our passions helps to act as our rudder and give us direction in flight and in life.

So, though we typically associate "yoga" with just the physical poses or meditation, you now know there is so much more. Yoga should not just be practiced on the yoga mat, in a yoga class, though that may be where it starts. Our lives should be based on being a good and moral person, practicing the 8 limbs of physical yoga to help guide us and give us direction in life. Taking our yoga off the yoga mat and into our daily lives involves selfless actions, faith, and continued study; practicing all four paths of yoga.

What does Om mean?

"Om" (also Ohm or Aum) is the divine sound of the universe. We are all just bodies of energy, and it is said if all the sounds of the universe were blended together, the sound would be Om. Om is often chanted at the beginning of a yoga class to bring the energies of the students together before practicing.

The sound of Om is broken down into three sounds. "A," "U," and "M." "A" represents our walking state, the earth and our past. We make this sound by opening our mouths saying "ahh." The "U" is our dream state, the mind, the middle, the present; encompassing everything and every sound. We make this sound by rounding our lips into a large O, with the tongue in the middle of the mouth, not touching the sides or top.

The "M" is our deep sleep state, our future and our heaven. The "M" sound is made by pressing the lips together and humming, the teeth stay apart and the tongue still does not touch the inside of the mouth. Feel the hum and vibration travel throughout your body.

The symbol for Om resembles the number 3 with a tail, a curve, and a dot to the right. The "A" (walking state) is represented at the lower curve of the 3 and the "M" (heavenly state) is the upper curve. The "O" (dream state) is represented by a line that resembles a tail and begins in the middle of the 3, but does not touch it, outside of reality, but present. The upper curve represents infinity and the dot represents the higher power (the one, the self, the Lord), separated from our earthly being, but ever present.

Why do people chant during yoga?

Chanting develops our concentration and strength of mind and helps purify negative emotions. When we chant, the sound produced by the body is absorbed into the mind and helps clear the mind of distractions. Chanting in groups can be empowering and raise the energy levels in a room, and is, therefore, sometimes chanted at the beginning or end of a yoga class. Chanting can also be silent. The sound of Om (Aum) can be chanted anywhere or anytime. Take a deep breath in through your nose and only exhale one-third of the breath as you chant "A" in your mind, exhale the second third and chant "U," finish the exhale with "M." Follow with one full inhale "Om," feeling energy rise from the base of the spine to the top of the head.

What is a mantra?

A mantra is a word or phrase that is repeated over and over again. By repeating a mantra aloud or in our minds, it begins to penetrate our energy cells, connecting our thoughts with our physical body. It can be a positive thought, intention, or sound, maybe "I am happy," "I am healthy," or "Om." I am sure you have heard of the concept, "the power of positive thinking," or to "visualize" a particular outcome, to help it become a reality. This positive thought can enter our being and enable our words and actions to be consistent with that desired outcome. If you want something to change in your life, especially an attitude or feeling, repeat that positive statement to yourself many times over. Write it on a piece of paper and place it in your wallet, read it every day. Write it on your bathroom mirror and say it every day. Think of a tune, and sing your mantra every day. Let those words enter every cell of your body, so it becomes reality.

What is a mudra?

A mudra is simply a hand position. You may see yoga pictures with the hands pressed together at the heart, this is called Anjali mudra or (Namasté hands). This hand position symbolizes a balancing of our "Hatha Yoga," the balance of the sun and masculine energy of the left side of our body, with the moon and feminine energy of the right side of our body. Allow the hands to gently touch, backing off with the dominant hand, thumbs at the center of the sternum and elbows softly resting at your sides. This mudra is often performed during a yoga class, at a moment when the students should draw their attention inward and sense the balance of their energies or as a salutation with the word "Namasté." Another hand position often seen, at least on magazine covers, is Jñana mudra (forefinger and thumb touching with remaining fingers extended). This mudra calms the nervous system and is used as a focusing tool. While in a seated pose, wrists can rest on the knees. The palms can face up for inspiration or to open awareness, or they can face down to calm the mind and help ground our intentions. This mudra is also useful when attempting a challenging balancing pose, to help focus the mind. There are many other hand positions in yoga, but these are the two most commonly seen.

What are the chakras (wheels of energy)?

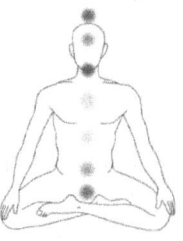

There are seven major areas where our nerves are bundled together along our spines. These nerves connect to our muscles and organs, and help control the flow of our subtle energies in the body affecting our nervous and endocrine systems. These seven areas are arranged vertically from the base of the spine to the top of the head and are called chakras or spinning "wheels of energy." As long as they keep spinning, our energy keeps flowing. Through life situations, our chakras can either be lacking in energy or have too much of it, and become imbalanced. The practice of yoga postures includes bends, twists, and movements of the spine in such a way as to keep the chakras open and spinning.

Our chakras are associated with the colors of the rainbow and have connections to our emotions, organs, and overall well-being. The root chakra is located at the base of the spine and is associated with the color red. This is our area for survival, food, shelter, love, and security. The belly chakra is orange and is located about 2 inches below the belly button. This is where we process pleasure and emotions. The solar plexus is in the stomach area, in the center of the body, and its color is yellow. Our solar plexus is our area for will, determination, and effort. The heart chakra is, of course, at the heart and associated with green. When our heart chakra is open and energy is flowing, we feel love, compassion, and joy. Next is the throat chakra, which is located in the throat, and is associated with blue; this is the area for truth and communication. The brow chakra (also called the "third eye") is indigo, on the forehead and between the eyebrows. This is our chakra for insight, imagination, and dreams. Lastly, is the crown chakra at the top of the head and the color is violet. This is where we connect with our spirituality and find true happiness.

Our energy travels upward from the base of the spine, so if you have heartburn and your heart chakra is "blocked" or still, the energy is not traveling to your throat for truthful communication or your mind for intuition. I like to compare our traveling energy to a visual of a slowly flowing pebble stream. Water pools into one area, spins and flows to the next pool, continuing down the stream. Now imagine if you put a rock in the way of the flowing water, blocking its path. The water would stop swirling in the pool, become still, and deprive the subsequent water pools of nourishment. Remove the rock and the water flows once again. Yoga postures work the various chakras and help keep the energy flowing from the root chakra to the crown chakra.

What does Namasté mean?

Namasté is a common greeting in the yoga world. There are long translations of the word but, essentially, it means "the goodness in me sees the goodness in you." It is about respecting the person you acknowledge, what they stand for, and who they are. We all have goodness in us, and it is nice when someone recognizes it.

At the end of a yoga class, most teachers will conclude with hands at heart center and with the word "Namasté" as a salutation to acknowledge the goodness of each person in the room. The students then return the greeting. I personally like to end my adult classes with the longer translation; "I honor the place in you where the universe resides. That place of love, light, honor, and truth. When you are in that place in you, and I am in that place in me, there is only one of us. Namasté."

Part 3 - YOGA CLASSES

Who can practice yoga?

Everyone. That is the beauty of yoga! Babies can do yoga (they already do), children can do yoga, grown-ups, and seniors too. No matter your age, body, or ability, there is a style and level of yoga you can do that will help you feel better physically, emotionally, and mentally. Talk with a certified yoga teacher to discuss any concerns you may have about beginning a yoga practice.

What are the benefits of practicing yoga?

Yoga has many physical benefits. Yoga can help improve strength; standing poses engage the large muscle groups of the legs and core. Using your own body weight, you can deepen lunges and engage muscle groups to intensify your practice. Yoga poses are also unique in that students may put weight onto their hands. Poses such as Downward Facing Dog improve upper body strength and prepare for more advanced arm balancing poses. It is important as we age to include weight-bearing exercises to maintain healthy bone density. Around age 20, we begin to lose our balance; but with practice, we can improve it one day at a time. Yoga not only has poses where you stand on one leg, it also focuses on the alignment of the joints, spine, and lift of the crown of the head; improving posture while balancing. Yoga also improves flexibility and encourages quicker results from the same stretches by incorporating awareness of the breath.

Internally, yoga improves digestion and helps oxygenate the organs through compression and twists. Through the various movements, the chakras (energy centers) are also engaged and internal energy flows more freely. Many yoga poses also stimulate the endocrine system, respiratory system, and circulatory system. Yoga also helps to lower blood pressure, improve mood, lessen back pain, reduce inflammation, and much more. There are books upon books with detailed yoga practices for improved health; *Yoga as Medicine, The Yogic Prescription for Health and Healing* by Timothy McCall, M.D., and *Dr. Yoga, A Complete Program for Discovering the Head-to-Toe Health Benefits of Yoga* by Nirmala Heriza, these are just a few great examples!

Mentally, yoga helps to calm the mind and body. Deep breathing not only improves lung capacity, it also calms the nervous system. Inverting the body (taking the head below the heart) is a naturally calming pose. Children naturally invert their bodies and love to be upside down, which oxygenates their brains and helps reset their moods. You don't see many adults hanging from the monkey bars, but certain yoga poses help invert the body to achieve similar benefits. (Inversions are not recommended for people with high blood pressure, glaucoma, or certain medical conditions. Consult your doctor before hanging from the monkey bars.)

Practicing the upper limbs of yoga (sense withdrawal, concentration and meditation) gives us mental strength to control the thoughts that occupy our mind. Our brain needs a break from all the chatter and it takes practice to learn to clear our minds. While balancing in a yoga pose, the mind is focused on not falling over and has an opportunity to practice the skill of steadiness. In more challenging yoga poses, keeping the breath and mind steady help prepare the body to handle stress in a calm way. Regular yoga practice helps the body keep stress levels low by calming the nervous system and training the body to handle stress in a more positive way.

What are the different styles of yoga?

Practicing postures (asana) is the 3rd limb of the 8-limbed Raja (yoga of action) yoga path. Most of the styles of yoga practiced in the West today are a form of Hatha Yoga. According to the original yoga texts, there are three purposes of Hatha Yoga: (1) purification of the body; (2) balance of the physical, mental, and energetic fields; and (3) awakening the pure consciousness by connecting with the divine. There are dozens of styles of Hatha Yoga with only slight variations. The majority of the poses are similar, but how they are taught and the emphasis of the class varies between them. A few examples of styles you might encounter…

- Anusara – is "heart oriented" and focuses on aligning with the divine in yoga and in daily life.

- Ashtanga Vinyasa – begins with Sun Salutations and continues through a set sequence of specific poses while moving with the breath.
- Bikram – is performed in a room heated to at least 105° and moves twice through a set series of 26 poses and 2 breathing exercises, named by leading teacher Bikram Choudhury.
- Iyengar – stresses alignment and perfecting poses with the use of props. Poses are held for long periods of time and named by leading teacher B.K.S. Iyengar.
- Kundalini – focuses on bringing energy to the body through deep rhythmic breathing, awakening the sleeping serpent (Kundalini) energy at the base of the spine.
- Power Yoga – is primarily drawn from the Ashtanga Vinyasa method and emphasizes a vigorous workout.
- Restorative – favors the use of props for supported poses. Poses are held for longer periods of time and are ideal for relaxation.
- Vinyasa flow – links postures with the breath. "Vin" means the wind, your breath. Poses are "placed in a special way."
- Yin Yoga – targets connective tissues, ligaments, and joints by holding seated postures for 2-5 minutes.

Which style of yoga should I practice?

Good question. Just like finding the right yoga teacher, you will need to experiment to find the right style of yoga class for you. Most athletes gravitate towards the hot and powerful classes which provide similar training to their bodies. My challenge to you would be to determine what level of activity you currently do, what your strengths are and help create balance in your physical and mental training. For the go-getter, it will be very challenging for them to sit and hold stretching poses for 2-5 minutes in a Yin yoga class, but that is also their mental training. Runners develop very tight leg muscles from repetitive training of the legs. Yin yoga would be a great balance for runners, helping their bodies be more efficient at using energy with more supple muscles. A dancer who can do the splits would benefit most from a more powerful class to help balance their flexibility and strength. Becoming a more efficient athlete requires balance in the body. A teacher once told me "a balanced body is a painless body." It is our job to find that balance in our physical training, as well as our personal and professional lives. Classes that blend a little bit of everything, like Vinyasa flow classes, are great for everyone; improving strength, flexibility, balance, and endurance.

What do I need for a yoga class?

First, you will need a sticky yoga mat (not an exercise mat, which will slip on typical wooden studio floors). Some studios and gyms have them available to use or to rent, but for hygienic reasons, it is recommended you bring your own. There are many kinds available, and most major retailers have inexpensive options. If you are looking for a high quality mat, ask your local studio. Some examples are Jade, Manduka, or Lululemon. If you have sensitive knees, you may wish to bring a small blanket or towel to place under your knees for extra cushion. Other props you may wish to bring (or may be available for you to use) might include a yoga strap, yoga block, or bolster.

If you are practicing hot yoga or tend to sweat a lot, I suggest you invest in a yoga mat towel to place on top of your yoga mat during class to prevent slipping and absorb perspiration. They typically have a non-slip back so they stay put on your mat and are easy to wash after a hot and sweaty class. You should dress comfortably and be able to move freely without wardrobe distraction; avoid buttons, zippers, and excessively baggy clothes. You may also want to remove jewelry and pull long hair back.

Is there yoga class etiquette?

Absolutely!! First and foremost, be on time for class, or, better yet, arrive early. One of the initial limbs of yoga is not to steal, "only take what is yours." This applies to other people's time as well. Depending on the studio environment, keep voices low and be respectful. Do not bring valuables to class. Take your shoes off and place them in the appropriate location. Turn your cell phone off (not just on vibrate) and put it away; do not take it to your mat and do not take pictures with your phone during a yoga class. During a quiet moment, the buzz…buzz…buzz… of a vibrating phone can be very distracting to students. You might also wonder if it is your phone, who is calling, what they need, etc. Give yourself permission to be digitally disconnected for one hour. Whatever it is, it can wait!!

Quietly set up your yoga mat, then take a seat or lie down. Different studios have different energies and regular students have their routines. Some take the opportunity to say hello to friends and others utilize quiet time before class to prepare their minds and bodies. In time, you will develop your own routine. During typical yoga classes, there is no dialogue between teacher and student. There may be an occasional joke (at least in my classes) or the teacher may approach an individual with a specific question asked quietly ("are you comfortable?") But as a rule of thumb, students do not blurt out questions or comments during class. Save your questions for after class and the teacher will be happy to answer them.

Do not chew gum or eat during a yoga class. You may be permitted to bring a water bottle to your mat, especially for a hot and sweaty yoga class, but be mindful it is not in the way of the teacher or your neighbor. If you have a tendency to sweat during class and your perspiration puddles on the floor, bring an extra hand towel to wipe it up. Puddles on the floor can be very dangerous as students pack up to leave class.

One of the moral disciplines is to "be pure." Clean yourself and your mat regularly. Avoid wearing lotions as they can make the hands, feet, and skin slippery as you begin to perspire. Do not wear strong perfumes or colognes, people are breathing deeply and may be sensitive to particular scents.

Lastly, do not leave a yoga class during relaxation time. If you have to leave class early due to another commitment, notify the teacher before class. Before final relaxation, roll up your mat, grab your belongings, and, as quietly as possible, exit the room. For many students, this is the only time of the day they get to just relax and let go, deepening their yoga practice. Going back to our principle of "do not steal," do not take this precious time from the other students in the class.

Why is yoga practiced barefoot?

The feet have tiny receptors on the bottom of them. When our shoes and socks are off, we can feel the earth beneath our feet. Practicing yoga with bare feet also helps improve balance. Our feet are often stuck in shoes during the day and we are not working the muscles of our feet. So kick off your shoes and try to pick up something small off of the floor, notice those muscles. In yoga, you become aware of the toes and feet and how they play a part in balance. Don't worry if your toes are not cute; no one is looking. And remember, there is no judgment in yoga, not even of yourself. Your toes are lovely; let them breathe!

How long are yoga classes?

Most yoga classes are about one hour in length. There are definitely classes that are an abbreviated version and only 30-45 minutes (often added onto another workout or as a lunchtime class). But that won't really give enough time to hold stretches or focus on the relaxation aspects of yoga, just enough for the body to feel better from movement and breathing exercises. Classes with longer holds for stretching or relaxation (Yin or Restorative) are often at least 90 minutes. However, do not let your time availability get in the way of practicing yoga. 5-10 minutes of yoga every day is far more beneficial than only one 60-minute class per week. When you feel your mind or body could use a break, do a little yoga. Yoga can be practiced anytime, anywhere, and for any length of time.

How long do I wait after eating before practicing yoga?

A general guideline is to wait two to three hours after a big meal and about one hour after a snack before practicing yoga. Yoga classes typically involve twists and inversions, and, unless you like heartburn or want to taste your food again, time your meals and classes appropriately.

Are all yoga teachers the same?

Finding the right yoga teacher reminds me of the story of Goldilocks and the Three Bears. Every teacher has their own style of delivering a yoga class. The pace at which they teach, the music they play (if any), the instructions or modifications they give, and the variety of content varies from teacher to teacher. Some teachers have a passion or a mission and they use their yoga class to expose and educate others to their passion. One teacher might teach too fast, another too slow; but just like Goldilocks, keep trying and you will eventually find the one that is just right for you! Once you find a teacher you love, it will change you forever!

Would I benefit from a private yoga session?

If you have any concerns about beginning a yoga practice, you might want to start with a private session. A certified yoga teacher can teach you basic yoga poses and help you get comfortable with terminology, alignment, and modifications for taking a group class. If you are concerned about looking silly or being embarrassed, private sessions can help you gain some experience and build confidence (though there is no judgment in yoga and that includes not judging ourselves either). After a few sessions, you should have the tools to attend a group class and feel comfortable with basic yoga poses and breathing exercises.

Private sessions are also great for those who are unable to travel to a studio, have a specific need or desired result, or prefer a particular pace of class. Private settings also allow the teacher to physically assist in pose positioning and help the student discover a deeper understanding of how poses should feel, versus how they look. To learn some yoga basics, visit TinyTurtleYoga.com, or to find a certified yoga instructor in your area visit YogaAlliance.org and search their directory.

Why do some yoga students use props?

There are many different props students can use to help them modify, intensify, or receive assistance in a yoga pose. A block, for example, can be used under your hands in a forward fold, if you are unable to reach the floor and desire support. While lying on the floor, a strap can be used (on the bottom of the foot) as an extension of the arm for a more comfortable hamstring stretch. Other props may include bolsters, blankets, chairs, or even the wall. Props can also help a student go deeper into a pose, so don't think of them as cheating or only for beginners, props are great for all levels! Many props can be purchased at Tiny Turtle Yoga's online store!

Do I need to be flexible to practice Yoga?

The answer is simple, No. Who better to attend a yoga class than someone who wants to improve their flexibility? Though not the purpose of yoga, it is a natural side effect! Regular yoga practice can improve flexibility through yoga poses, which both strengthen and stretch the muscles. Through yoga breathing, your muscles receive more oxygen, making the stretches more effective. The muscles should be warmed up with yoga poses that engage the large muscle groups like Sun Salutations or Warrior Poses. While holding stretches, breathing deeply sends more oxygen to the muscles, allowing them to elongate slowly like taffy. Avoid cold, short bursts of tension on the muscle (ballistic stretching) because bouncing or pushing may tear the muscle instead of stretching it. Sensation while stretching is good; but pain is not. Never force the muscles of the body to stretch past their current limits; it is a slow process and it will take time to get the most out of practicing yoga. To quote Kathryn Budig, one of my favorite yoga teachers, "You will only be a beginner once, so enjoy the journey!"

How is yoga breathing different from my normal breath?

The majority of yoga breathing is done through the nose. The nose has a natural filtration system that enables the air we breathe through our nose to be cleaner than the air we breathe through our mouth.

Pranayama (breath control) is the fourth limb on the yoga tree. Prana means "vital energy", and yama means "to control." The nasal passages are also linked with our energy system. Through breath control, we can balance and regulate vital energy in our bodies. When we control breath and energy, we control our mind. Breathing in is called an "inhalation" and draws the energy of the universe into the body. Breathing out is an "exhalation" and removes toxins from the system, providing room for energy to exist and expand. As you have learned, we have different energies. Try this little experiment; use one finger to close off one side of your nose and breathe, now try the other side. For most people, one side will be "more open" than the other side; this is your current dominant energy. If your left nostril was more open, your moon energy, creative, and calm side is more active right now. If your right nostril was more open, your masculine, logic, and active side is more active. If both sides were relatively the same, your energies are balanced and focused, the optimal state for learning and problem solving. Breathing exercises can help balance our energies for our desired result; to help us calm, energize, or focus the mind and body.

Most people only use one-third of their lung capacity, which is observed when only the upper chest is moving while breathing, called "chest breathing." This breath is short and shallow and leaves the body in a constant "startled state." To see where you breathe, you can place one hand on your upper chest and the other just below your belly button and see which one is moving when you inhale. If you watch a baby breathe, their belly rises and falls, while their rib cage remains relatively still. As we age, we have a tendency to "suck it in," shift our breathing to our chest and stop moving our bellies when we breathe. The first step to deepening the breath is to practice relaxed diaphragmatic breathing; deep, smooth, even breaths, without sound or pause. Lie on the floor, and place the hands back on the chest and belly. Now breathe deeply into the belly, allowing that hand to rise, and fill the lungs as much as you can. This breath has three parts. It begins in the low belly, moves up to the chest, and then the belly and chest move together. Slowly exhale completely until the belly button sinks towards the spine, relax the muscles of the abdomen and repeat. Focus on your breath, in and out. This deep breathing will trigger the relaxation response in the body and provide more oxygen to your muscles and organs.

While in a yoga class, you may hear other students breathing rather loudly. This audible breath is called Ujjayi (you-jie-ee) breathing or "Vader breath." To create this sounding breath, inhale and exhale out of the mouth, onto your hand, like you are fogging a mirror. Notice the breath is moist and warm. This constriction of the glottis soothes the nerves and calms the mind. Maintaining that constriction, the Ujjayi breath is a "ha" whisper out of the nose on the exhale, and an "ah" on the inhale (which sounds similar to the breathing of Darth Vader in *Star Wars*). This breath often sounds like ocean waves in your head, guiding you through your yoga practice. If you are listening to your breath and notice it becomes shallow, jagged, or still during a yoga class, it may suggest you have gone too far or need a break. After reestablishing slow, smooth breaths again, resume your yoga practice with more awareness of your breath.

As your body works harder in a yoga pose, continue to breathe steadily, keeping the nervous system calm. You are training your body to handle stress in a relaxed manner. As you go through life and encounter difficult situations, your body will remember how to respond; maintain slow steady breaths and help reduce stress levels.

How can yoga help me reduce stress?

Many yoga poses are naturally calming. Taking slow, deep, full breaths can help relax the mind and body; forward folds and inversions (head below the heart) are also calming for most people, relaxing the nervous system and counteracting the effects of stress. People typically react to stress in one of three ways; they get angry and agitated, quiet and withdrawn, or they shut down. How do you respond to stress? Once you know this, you will be better able to identify which type of yoga to practice to specifically reduce the stress in your body. You probably already have something you do when you need to de-stress (go for a walk, call a friend, paint, etc.). This can be a clue as to what your body needs. If you react by getting angry, your body is in a heightened state of agitation; you need deep breaths, calming poses, and stretching to help bring the body and mind back to the present. If you withdraw or shut down, active poses that engage the mind and body will be more effective; flowing poses, strengthening poses, and energizing breaths can help. Lastly, if you have a tendency to just shut down and go blank, you need to reboot! Get up, get moving, breathe, oxygenate, and reset the body system. You may be clearly in one category or more of a combination. This too may require some experimentation to find out which yoga techniques help you manage your stress most effectively.

What do the yoga certifications mean?

Yoga education and training was traditionally passed down from guru (or master) to student. They worked closely together for many years until the guru felt the student was ready to teach another. As yoga came west and gained in popularity, there needed to be a standard of education and proof of certification. Yoga Alliance developed training guidelines for teachers and schools in 1999. Qualified yoga teachers should hold a minimum of a Registered Yoga Teacher (RYT-200) certification. After many years of experience, they earn the designation Experienced Registered Yoga Teacher (ERYT).

RYT 200 – completed 200 hours of training

RYT 500 – completed 500 hours of training and 100 hours of teaching experience

ERYT 200 – completed 200 hours of training and 1,000 hours of teaching experience

ERYT 500 – completed 500 hours of training and 2,000 hours of teaching experience

RCYT (Registered Children's Yoga Teacher) – completed an additional 95 hours of training for children's yoga, 30 hours teaching children

RPYT (Registered Prenatal Yoga Teacher) – completed an additional 85 hours of training for prenatal yoga, 30 hours teaching prenatal yoga

Why do people get hurt while practicing yoga?

Having a well-trained teacher is very important. Yoga teachers should be Registered Yoga Teachers (RYT) through Yoga Alliance, verifying they completed the proper amount of training to teach yoga, offer modifications, and help keep their students safe. You can find a qualified teacher near you through their online directory YogaAlliance.org.

Having proper instruction is key. Even the best athlete should start with a beginners' yoga class or introductory workshop, building a foundation and learning the fundamentals of form and alignment. If yoga were like a math class, you would not jump right into calculus without learning algebra first. Attending a difficult class or doing challenging poses does not necessarily classify a student as more advanced. The advanced practitioner is one who can slow down, appreciate the subtleties of poses, and listen to their body.

Yoga class is non-judgmental and non-competitive, but in such a competitive world, it is a difficult concept for new students to accept. If another student is doing the most advanced variation of a pose, they want to try it too, despite the fact they do not know how to safely enter, execute, or exit the pose. The best thing to do is ask the teacher after class how to prepare the body to do the more advanced pose and get instruction on how to do it safely. Letting go of ego is one of the most challenging aspects of yoga, especially for competitive athletes. Sensation is good, but pain is bad. There is no pain in yoga. If your body senses pain (especially in the joints), it is telling you to stop before you get injured. Your body is having a conversation with you; be on the receiving end of that conversation, listen and respond.

Lastly, if you have a preexisting injury or special condition, inform your teacher before class. They can offer modifications and keep an eye on you during class. Your yoga teacher should guide you to choose the best variation of poses to suit your personal needs. You do not want to leave a yoga class feeling worse than when you arrived. You want to feel better. Practice compassion and acceptance with your body; it is the only one you get!

What can I expect to do during a Yoga class?

Some yoga classes may begin with chanting the word "Om," to help bring the energies of the room together, followed by a warm up to loosen the body and prepare it to do more challenging poses. A variation of a Sun Salutation is often practiced but, depending on the level of the class, the instructor may choose other poses to warm the muscles and joints. During a yoga class, you will typically encounter a variety of categories of poses including seated poses, standing poses, forward folds, back bends, twists, balance poses, core work, inversions, and restorative poses. There should be a balance between strengthening and stretching poses, forward folds and back bends, as well as a balance between poses on the left and right. A well-choreographed sequence will prepare your body for the more advanced poses you might see towards the end of the class and leave you feeling relaxed, comfortable, and alert. Classes typically end with 5-15 minutes of relaxation, often in Savasana (or Corpse Pose). It is during final relaxation that students begin to practice concentration and meditation.

Why do yogis look like they are sleeping at the end of class?

At the end of most yoga classes, there is time for final relaxation, often in Savasana (Corpse Pose). Despite what it looks like, it is not a time to sleep. After a yoga class, students have practiced many of the limbs of the yoga tree. It is now time for them to advance to the final limbs of sense withdrawal, concentration, and mediation. It is a time to be super conscious (not unconscious), completely aware, but detached from the surroundings; a time to listen to their breath and find the space between thoughts that is quiet and still. It is during relaxation that the body absorbs the benefits of yoga. During a yoga class, the body creates energy and does not transfer it to another object like when a ball is kicked. This energy continues to travel through the body and, during relaxation pose, the energy can penetrate the cells of the body and repair damaged cells. If the body moves, that energy is used for the movement. If a thought arises, that energy is used for the thought. The challenge is to remain still, silent, and completely relaxed. The relaxation pose is probably one of the most challenging poses for adults to learn but, with regular practice, they learn to love it!

What is the purpose of guided visualizations?

In today's busy world, we have a hard time detaching from the daily grind and our minds are constantly working. Some teachers lead their students through guided visualizations at the end of a yoga class, helping to focus the students' minds on something else. In these moments, we are not thinking about errands, bills, work, or relationships. Instead, the mind is given permission to focus on something else, something calming and peaceful, possibly inspiring or enlightening. If you have a place you find especially relaxing, like the beach, find guided visualizations which take place at the beach. As with everything yoga, it takes practice. Start with a short visualization, maybe only a few minutes, and gradually add more time as you get more comfortable. If your mind wanders during a visual exercise and you think of something else, that is okay. Just acknowledge that it was there, without judgment, and refocus on the visualization. This focused relaxation allows the whole body and mind to let go and reset. Finding deep relaxation of mind and body for only twenty minutes can be rejuvenating and energizing; this is equivalent to about a two-hour nap!

How often should I practice yoga?

If you are practicing yoga as your main method of exercise, it is recommended that you raise your heart rate for at least 30 minutes, three times a week. If you are practicing yoga as a way to balance other workouts, plan yoga classes in between workouts, but be mindful not to push the same muscle groups day after day, they need time to recover. I hope you now know that there are many different styles and intensities of yoga. Maybe one day is focused on strengthening, another day on stretching. If you are sore from a yoga class, attend another one 24 hours later and work on stretching your sore muscles. Your body needs time to recover between intense workouts.

However, yoga can be practiced every day. A little bit of yoga every day can be extremely beneficial and rewarding. Five to ten minutes of deep breathing or a few simple twists and stretches before bedtime is a great way to incorporate yoga into your daily routine. As with anything, know your limits and listen to your body. Gradually build your personal practice to help create physical and mental balance.

Can I practice yoga at home?

There are many great DVDs, television programs, and online resources to enable you to add yoga to your day in the comfort of your own home. I practice at home with a monthly subscription to YogaGlo.com. This is a great way to get familiar with yoga poses, terminology, and gain confidence. However, in addition to practicing at home, I would suggest also attending group yoga classes with a certified teacher. You will find the energy in a live class is motivating and encouraging, helping you to feel the emotional benefits of yoga, as well as the physical ones. It is also a good idea to have a qualified teacher observe your practice, to provide cues and suggestions to help you modify, intensify, or safely execute postures (you don't want to develop bad habits that might lead to injury). Find balance in practicing both at home and at a yoga studio; try to practice a little bit of yoga every day.

When should I start practicing yoga?

Today!! Right now!! Stand up tall and take a few deep breaths. Reach your arms up over your head, interlace your fingers, and press your palms to the sky; add a little side bend to the left and to the right. Place your hands on the back of your hips, look up and begin to lift your heart in a gentle backbend. Now bend your knees, and fold forward from the hips. Allow your head to hang low, shake it a little "yes" and a little "no." Now gently roll your body back up to standing, one vertebrae at a time! Congratulations, you just did yoga!

Tiny Turtle Yoga:

TinyTurlteYoga.com

FREE Yoga Guide to Energy Strategies for Kids

Tiny Turtle Yoga Videos

Tiny Turtle Yoga Online Store

The Learning Station (http://www.learningstationmusic.com)

Suggested Resources:

- *YogaKids: Educating the Whole Child Through Yoga* by Marsha Wenig
- *Yoga as Medicine, The Yogic Prescription for Health and Healing* by Timothy McCall, M.D.
- *Dr. Yoga, A Complete Program for Discovering the Head-to-Toe Health Benefits of Yoga* by Nirmala Heriza
- *The Women's Health: Big Book of Yoga, The Essential Guide to Complete Mind/Body Fitness* by Kathryn Budig
- *Teaching Yoga: Essentials, Foundations and Techniques* by Mark Stephens
- *Guiding Yoga's Light: Lessons for Yoga Teachers* by Nancy Gerstein
- *Yoga: Mastering the Basics* by Sandra Anserson and Rolf Sovik
- YogaAlliance.org
- YogaKids.com
- YogaGlo.com